I0774345

HEMOCHROMATOSIS COOKBOOK

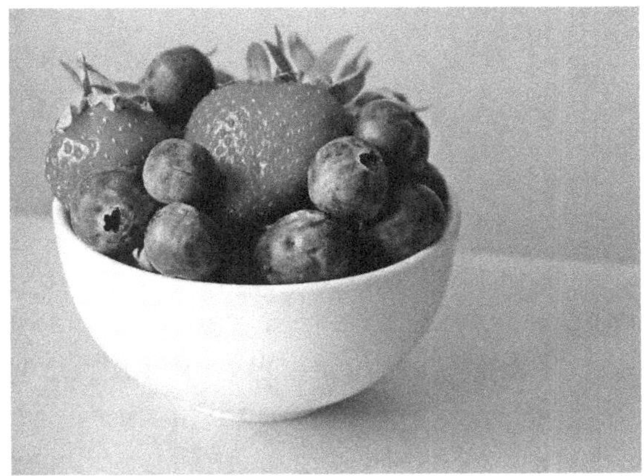

A complete recipes and meal prep for reducing the
absorption of iron in your diet

Avila Wanda

Table of content

Table of content   3

Introduction   5

Chapter one   7

  Meaning of hemochromatosis   7

Chapter two   11

  Other causes of hemochromatosis   11

Chapter three   15

  Symptoms of hemochromatosis   15

Chapter four   19

  Why do humans need iron   19

Chapter five   23

  How much iron is recommended every day   23

    So what are the foods that contains iron   25

Chapter six   29

  Diagnosis of hemochromatosis   29

Chapter seven   35

  Treatment of hemochromatosi   35

Chapter eight   41

  The hemochromatosis diets   41

Chapter nine   47

  Beneficial foods   47

Chapter ten   53

  Foods to avoid and a shopping list for
hemochromatosis   53

    Foods to Avoid in Hemochromatosis: 53

    Hemochromatosis-Friendly Shopping List:
55

Chapter eleven   59

Meal plan and time table for hemochromatosis 59

Sample Meal Plan: 59

Tips for Hemochromatosis Meal Planning:61

Chapter twelve **65**

Soups and Salads 65

Soups: 65

Salads: 66

Tips for Hemochromatosis-Friendly Soups and Salads: 68

Chapter thirteen **71**

Desserts 71

1. Fruit Salad with Mint: 71

2. Yogurt Parfait: 72

3. Chia Seed Pudding: 72

4. Sorbet: 73

5. Baked Apples: 74

6. Banana Nice Cream: 75

Tips for Hemochromatosis-Friendly Desserts: 75

Conclusion **77**

Introduction

In the bustling world of culinary exploration, where flavors dance and ingredients harmonize, there emerges a unique endeavor – the Hemochromatosis Cookbook. As the pages unfold, it unveils a narrative interwoven with the delicate balance between health and gastronomy.

In this culinary odyssey, the protagonist is not a conventional hero but a condition – hemochromatosis. A genetic disorder that causes the body to absorb and store excessive iron, hemochromatosis necessitates a mindful approach to nutrition. The cookbook is an indispensable guide for those navigating this journey, offering a symphony of recipes tailored to meet the specific dietary needs of individuals managing this condition.

Within the cookbook's pages, each recipe is a testament to the creative fusion of taste and health. From hearty entrees to delectable desserts, the collection is a celebration of culinary diversity that accommodates the constraints imposed by hemochromatosis. It transforms the kitchen into a haven where one can relish delicious meals without compromising well-being.

Moreover, the Hemochromatosis Cookbook transcends the boundaries of a mere recipe compendium; it becomes a companion, offering not just sustenance but a holistic approach to living with hemochromatosis. The introduction sets the stage for a journey where ingredients become allies, and flavors are curated with precision to embrace a life of vitality and taste.

For those touched by the nuances of hemochromatosis, this cookbook becomes more than just a guide; it is a narrative of resilience, a culinary testament to the art of savoring life even in the face of unique health challenges.

Chapter one

Meaning of hemochromatosis

Hemochromatosis is a hereditary disorder characterized by an excessive accumulation of iron in the body. Typically, the body tightly regulates iron absorption to maintain balance, but individuals with hemochromatosis absorb and store too much iron, leading to potential complications.

This genetic condition primarily stems from mutations in the HFE gene, affecting the body's ability to regulate iron absorption from the digestive system. The most common form of hereditary hemochromatosis is caused by mutations in the HFE gene, particularly the C282Y and H63D variants.

As iron builds up over time, it deposits in various organs such as the liver, heart, pancreas, and joints, potentially causing damage and dysfunction. Symptoms may not manifest until later stages when iron overload has already occurred. Common signs include fatigue, joint pain, abdominal pain, and skin discoloration.

One of the concerning aspects of hemochromatosis is its potential to lead to serious complications if left untreated. Organ damage, particularly to the liver (cirrhosis) and heart, can result in life-threatening conditions. Additionally, the increased iron levels may contribute to diabetes, arthritis, and hormonal imbalances.

Diagnosis often involves blood tests to assess iron levels, transferrin saturation, and genetic testing for HFE mutations. Treatment primarily revolves around phlebotomy, a process similar to blood donation, aimed at reducing iron levels in the body. Regular monitoring and management help individuals with hemochromatosis lead healthy lives.

Understanding the implications of hemochromatosis involves recognizing the delicate balance of iron in the body and the potential consequences when this equilibrium is disrupted due to genetic factors. Timely detection and appropriate management are essential to mitigate the risks associated with iron overload in individuals affected by this condition.

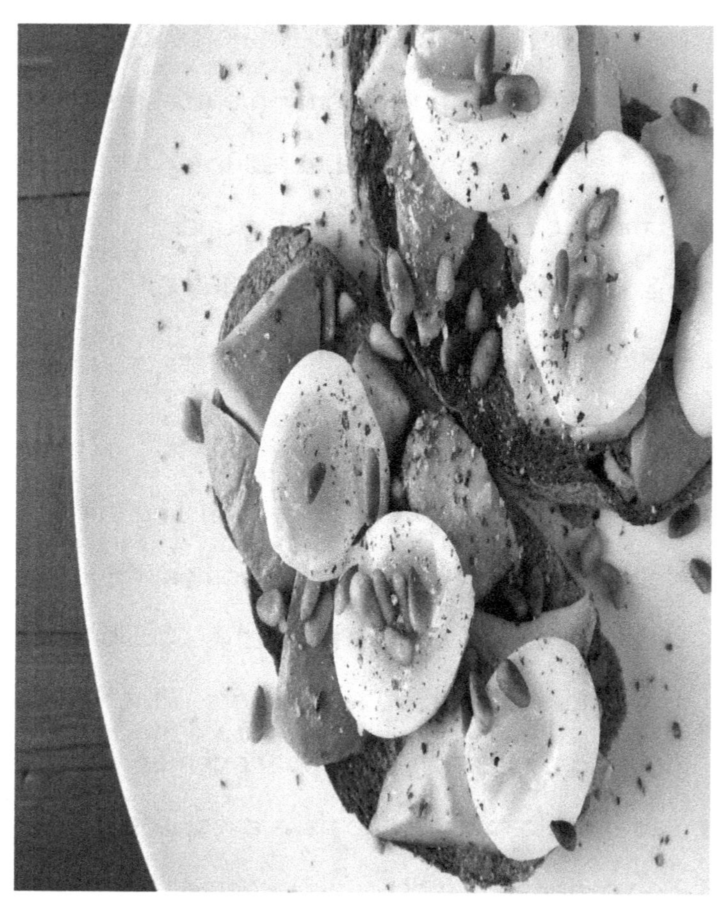

Chapter two

Other causes of hemochromatosis

While hereditary hemochromatosis, primarily linked to mutations in the HFE gene, is the most common form, there are other causes of hemochromatosis that are not related to genetics. These non-genetic forms are often referred to as secondary or acquired hemochromatosis. Here are some notable causes:

1. Iron Overload Disorders: Certain medical conditions, such as thalassemia and other types of anemia, can lead to increased iron absorption and subsequent overload. In these cases, the excessive iron is a result of the

body's response to chronic blood transfusions.

2. Chronic Liver Diseases: Conditions like alcoholic liver disease, nonalcoholic fatty liver disease (NAFLD), and chronic hepatitis C can cause liver damage, leading to disruptions in iron regulation and accumulation.

3. Excessive Iron Intake: In rare cases, excessive consumption of iron supplements or prolonged intravenous iron therapy can result in iron overload.

4. African Iron Overload: Also known as Bantu siderosis, this condition is prevalent in certain African populations. It is associated with the traditional dietary practice of cooking in iron pots, leading to elevated iron levels.

5. Porphyria Cutanea Tarda (PCT): This is
   a rare form of porphyria that can be
   associated with iron overload. PCT
   affects the skin and may lead to
   increased iron absorption.
6. Repeated Blood Transfusions:
   Individuals who receive frequent blood
   transfusions, such as those with certain
   blood disorders like sickle cell disease,
   thalassemia, or myelodysplastic
   syndromes, can accumulate excess iron
   over time.

Diagnosing the specific cause of
hemochromatosis involves a thorough medical
evaluation, including a detailed patient history,
blood tests, and sometimes liver biopsy. The
treatment approach may vary depending on
the underlying cause but often involves

phlebotomy or iron-chelating medications to reduce iron levels in the body. Understanding the diverse causes of hemochromatosis is crucial for accurate diagnosis and effective management.

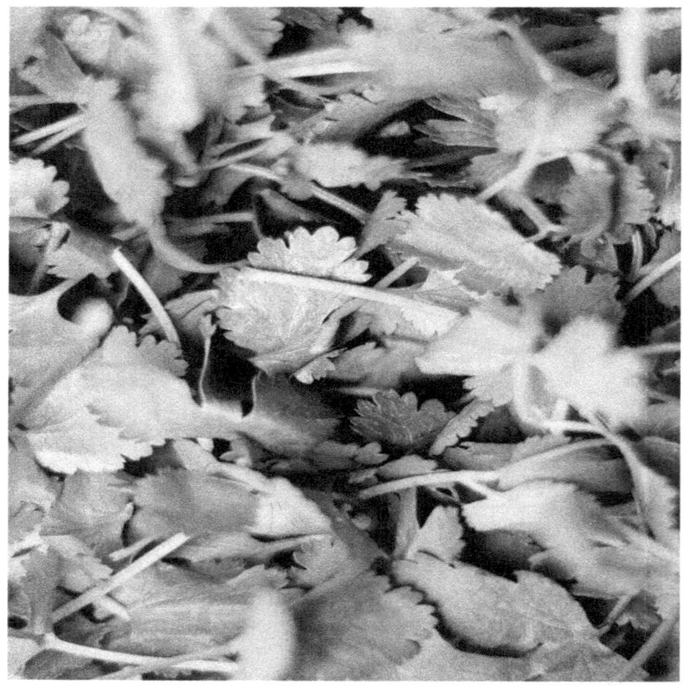

Chapter three

Symptoms of hemochromatosis

Hemochromatosis symptoms can be subtle in the early stages, and individuals may not experience noticeable effects until iron levels have become significantly elevated. Common symptoms of hemochromatosis include:

1. Fatigue: Persistent fatigue and weakness are often early indicators of hemochromatosis. The excess iron in the body can affect energy levels and overall vitality.

2. Joint Pain: Iron accumulation in the joints can lead to pain, stiffness, and discomfort. Arthritis-like symptoms, particularly in the hands and knuckles, are common.

3. Abdominal Pain: Iron overload can
    cause abdominal pain, often associated
    with an enlarged liver or spleen. This
    can result from iron deposition in these
    organs.

4. Skin Changes: A classic sign is bronze
    or grayish skin pigmentation, commonly
    referred to as "bronze diabetes." This
    discoloration is especially noticeable in
    areas with sun exposure.

5. Loss of Sex Drive: Hemochromatosis
    can impact hormonal balance, leading to
    a decreased libido and, in some cases,
    reproductive issues.

6. Weakness and Shortness of Breath: Iron
    accumulation in the heart can lead to
    cardiomyopathy, resulting in weakness
    and shortness of breath.

7. Diabetes: Iron overload may contribute to insulin resistance and diabetes, particularly in individuals with a genetic predisposition.

8. Liver Dysfunction: As iron accumulates in the liver, it can lead to conditions such as cirrhosis, which may manifest as abdominal pain, jaundice, and fluid retention.

9. Irregular Heartbeat: In severe cases, hemochromatosis can affect the electrical conduction system of the heart, leading to arrhythmias.

It's essential to note that not everyone with hemochromatosis will experience all of these symptoms, and the severity can vary widely. Moreover, some individuals may remain asymptomatic or show only mild symptoms.

Regular monitoring of iron levels, especially in individuals with a family history of hemochromatosis, is crucial for early detection and effective management of the condition. If symptoms are present or there's a concern about hemochromatosis, seeking medical advice and undergoing appropriate testing is recommended.

Chapter four

Why do humans need iron

The mineral iron is vital to human health because it is involved in many different physiological processes. Here are key reasons why humans need iron:

1. Oxygen Transport: Iron is a vital component of hemoglobin, the protein in red blood cells responsible for transporting oxygen from the lungs to tissues throughout the body. Hemoglobin binds with oxygen in the lungs, forms oxyhemoglobin, and releases oxygen in tissues as needed.

2. Cellular Respiration: Iron is also a component of myoglobin, a protein found in muscle cells that facilitates the

storage and release of oxygen for muscle contraction during physical activity.

3. Energy Production: Iron is involved in the electron transport chain within mitochondria, the cellular structures responsible for energy production. It plays a role in the synthesis of adenosine triphosphate (ATP), the primary energy currency of cells.

4. DNA Synthesis and Repair: Iron is crucial for the synthesis and repair of DNA, the genetic material in cells. It is involved in several enzymes that play essential roles in these processes.

5. Immune Function: Iron is necessary for the proper functioning of the immune system. It supports the activity of

immune cells and helps in the defense against infections.

While iron is vital for these functions, it's important to maintain a balance. Too little iron can lead to iron deficiency anemia, characterized by fatigue, weakness, and impaired cognitive function. On the other hand, excessive iron, as seen in conditions like hemochromatosis, can lead to toxicity and organ damage.

Dietary sources of iron include red meat, poultry, fish, beans, lentils, fortified cereals, and dark green leafy vegetables. In some cases, individuals may require iron supplements, especially if they have difficulty absorbing iron from their diet or have increased iron needs due to factors like pregnancy or growth during childhood. Balancing iron intake is crucial for overall health and well-being.

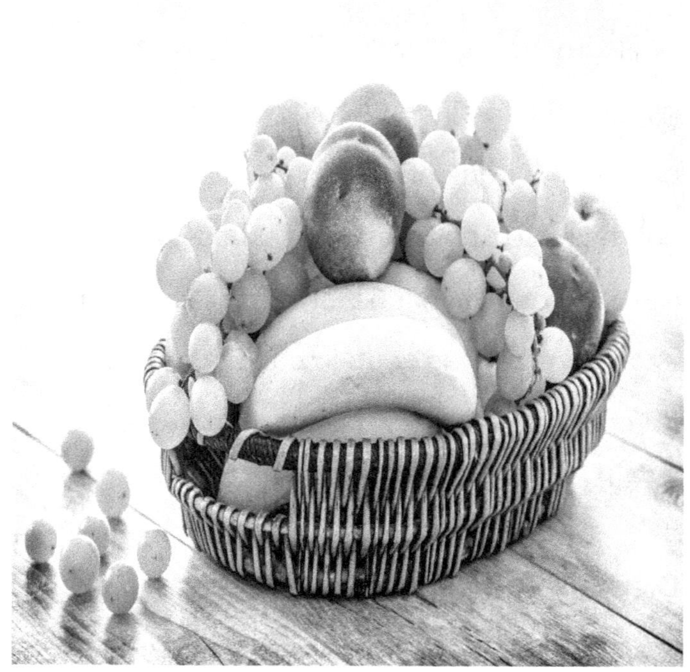

Chapter five

How much iron is recommended every day

The recommended daily intake of iron can vary based on factors such as age, sex, and life stage. The Recommended Dietary Allowance (RDA) for iron is expressed in milligrams (mg) per day. Here are the general recommendations:

1. Infants:
   - 0-6 months: 0.27 mg
   - 7-12 months: 11 mg
2. Children:
   - 1-3 years: 7 mg
   - 4-8 years: 10 mg
   - 9-13 years: 8 mg
3. Adolescents and Adults:

- o Males 14-18 years: 11 mg
- o Females 14-18 years: 15 mg
- o Males 19 years and older: 8 mg
- o Females 19-50 years: 18 mg
- o Females 51 years and older: 8 mg

4. Pregnant Women:
- o 14-18 years: 27 mg
- o 19 years and older: 27 mg

5. Breastfeeding Women:
- o 14-18 years: 10 mg
- o 19 years and older: 9 mg

It's important to note that iron recommendations can be influenced by factors such as dietary choices, absorption efficiency, and individual health conditions. Additionally, the form of iron found in food can affect absorption; heme iron (from animal sources) is more readily absorbed than non-heme iron (from plant sources).

Certain populations, such as pregnant women, growing children, and individuals with conditions like iron-deficiency anemia, may have higher iron requirements. Conversely, some individuals, like postmenopausal women and adult men, may require less iron.

So what are the foods that contains iron

Iron is present in various foods, and it's important to consume a balanced diet to meet your body's iron requirements. There are two main types of dietary iron: heme iron, found in animal products, and non-heme iron, found in plant and fortified foods. Examples of foods high in iron are as follows:

Heme Iron Sources (Animal Products):

1. Red Meat: Beef, lamb, and pork are rich sources of heme iron.
2. Poultry: Chicken and turkey provide heme iron.
3. Fish: Particularly, oily fish like salmon and tuna contain heme iron.

Non-Heme Iron Sources (Plant and Fortified Foods):

1. Legumes: Beans, lentils, chickpeas, and soybeans are good sources of non-heme iron.
2. Nuts and Seeds: Pumpkin seeds, sunflower seeds, almonds, and cashews contain iron.

3. Whole Grains: Foods like quinoa, fortified cereals, and oatmeal can contribute to iron intake.
4. Vegetables: Dark leafy greens such as spinach, kale, and Swiss chard are rich in non-heme iron.
5. Tofu and Tempeh: These plant-based protein sources also contain iron.
6. Dried Fruits: Prunes, apricots, and raisins are examples of dried fruits with iron.

Fortified Foods:

1. Fortified Cereals: Many breakfast cereals are fortified with iron.
2. Fortified Plant Milks: Some plant-based milk alternatives, like fortified almond or soy milk, can provide added iron.

To enhance iron absorption, consider pairing iron-rich foods with sources of vitamin C, such as citrus fruits, strawberries, or bell peppers. On the other hand, certain substances like calcium and tannins (found in tea and coffee) can inhibit iron absorption, so it's advisable to avoid consuming them with iron-rich meals.

Remember that individual iron needs can vary, and if you have specific concerns or dietary restrictions, it's recommended to consult with a healthcare professional or a registered dietitian to ensure you are meeting your nutritional requirements.

Chapter six

Diagnosis of hemochromatosis

Hemochromatosis diagnosis is made by combining genetic testing, laboratory testing, and clinical assessment. Here are key aspects of the diagnostic process for hemochromatosis:

1. Clinical Assessment:
   - Medical History: A thorough review of the patient's medical history, including any family history of hemochromatosis, symptoms, and risk factors.
   - Symptoms: Inquiring about symptoms associated with iron overload, such as fatigue, joint pain, abdominal pain, and skin changes.

2. Laboratory Tests:

   o Serum Iron Levels: Measurement
     of serum iron levels to assess the
     amount of iron circulating in the
     blood.

   o Transferrin Saturation (TSAT):
     Calculating the percentage of
     transferrin that is saturated with
     iron, providing information about
     iron transport.

   o Serum Ferritin: Ferritin is a
     protein that stores iron; elevated
     levels indicate increased iron
     stores in the body.

   o Complete Blood Count (CBC):
     Checking for anemia and other
     blood abnormalities associated
     with hemochromatosis.

3. Genetic Testing:

- HFE Gene Mutation Analysis:
    Genetic testing for mutations in
    the HFE gene, particularly the
    C282Y and H63D variants. The
    majority of hereditary
    hemochromatosis cases are
    linked to mutations in the HFE
    gene.
  - Other Genes: In some cases,
    additional genetic testing may be
    performed to identify mutations in
    other genes associated with
    non-HFE hemochromatosis.

4. Liver Biopsy (in some cases):
  - Assessment of Iron Levels in
    Liver Tissue: A liver biopsy may
    be recommended to directly
    measure the amount of iron in the
    liver. This procedure is less

commonly used today due to the availability of less invasive diagnostic methods.

5. Imaging Studies (in some cases):

   - MRI (Magnetic Resonance Imaging): Non-invasive imaging techniques, such as MRI, can be used to assess iron levels in the liver. This method is increasingly utilized as an alternative to liver biopsy.

Early detection is crucial in managing hemochromatosis effectively. Routine screening may be recommended, especially for individuals with a family history of the condition. Additionally, healthcare providers may consider genetic testing if symptoms or abnormal laboratory results suggest hemochromatosis. A multi-faceted approach, involving clinical evaluation, laboratory tests, and genetic analysis, helps ensure accurate diagnosis and timely intervention to prevent complications associated with iron overload.

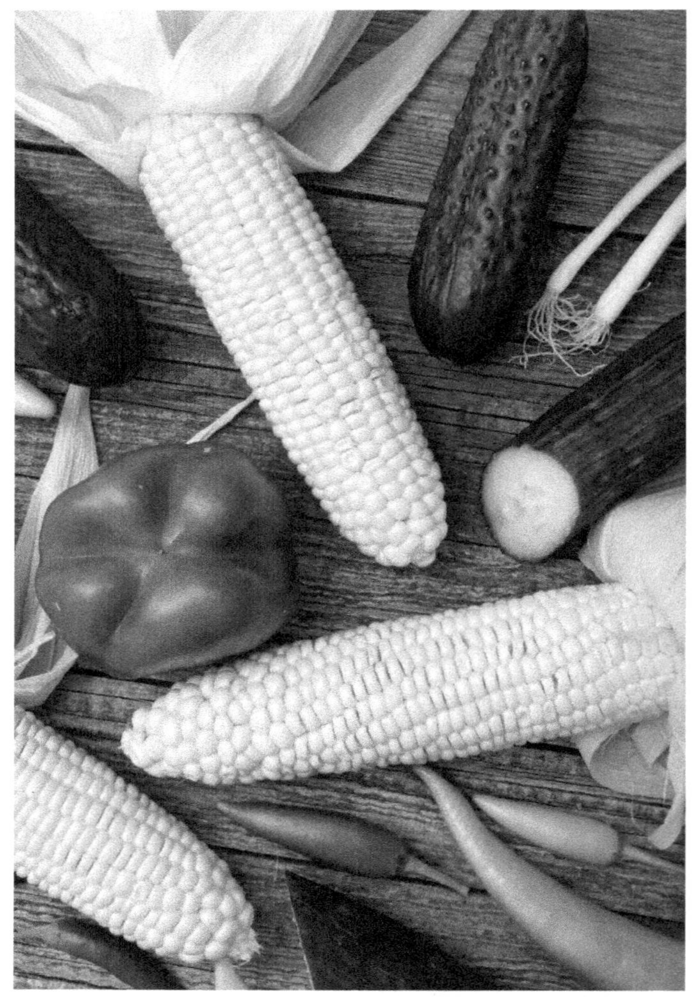

Chapter seven

Treatment of hemochromatosi

The primary goal of treating hemochromatosis is to reduce iron levels in the body to normal ranges, preventing organ damage and associated complications. Treatment approaches typically focus on the removal of excess iron and managing the underlying genetic or acquired causes. Here are key aspects of the treatment of hemochromatosis:

1. Phlebotomy (Blood Removal):
    - Primary Treatment Method: Phlebotomy is the most common and effective treatment for hereditary hemochromatosis. It involves the removal of a specific

amount of blood at regular intervals. This process lowers iron levels in the body over time.

- Frequency: Initially, phlebotomy sessions may be frequent (e.g., weekly), and the frequency is adjusted based on the individual's response and the rate of iron reduction.
- Maintenance: Once iron levels are within the normal range, maintenance phlebotomy is continued, typically at less frequent intervals (e.g., every few months).

2. Iron Chelation Therapy (in some cases):

- For Non-Responsive Cases: In individuals who cannot tolerate or do not respond well to phlebotomy, iron chelation therapy may be considered. Chelating agents, such as deferoxamine or deferasirox, bind to excess iron and facilitate its elimination from the body.

- Commonly Used in Secondary Hemochromatosis: Iron chelation therapy is more commonly employed in conditions leading to secondary iron overload, such as thalassemia or repeated blood transfusions.

3. Dietary Modifications:

- Reducing Iron Intake: Individuals with hemochromatosis are often advised to moderate their dietary iron intake. This may include limiting consumption of iron-rich foods and avoiding vitamin supplements containing iron.

- Avoiding Alcohol: As alcohol can exacerbate liver damage in individuals with hemochromatosis, limiting or avoiding alcohol consumption is recommended.

4. Monitoring and Follow-up:

- Regular Blood Tests: Continuous monitoring of iron levels, transferrin saturation, and ferritin levels helps assess the effectiveness of treatment and adjust interventions accordingly.
- Genetic Counseling: For individuals with hereditary hemochromatosis, genetic counseling is often recommended

to provide information about the condition, assess family risk, and discuss implications for family members.

5. Management of Complications:

   - Addressing Organ Damage: If complications such as liver cirrhosis or diabetes have already occurred, additional treatments or management strategies may be necessary.

Treatment plans are tailored to individual needs, considering factors like age, overall health, and the presence of complications. Early diagnosis and consistent management play a crucial role in preventing long-term consequences of hemochromatosis. It's important for individuals with hemochromatosis to work closely with healthcare professionals to develop and implement a comprehensive treatment plan.

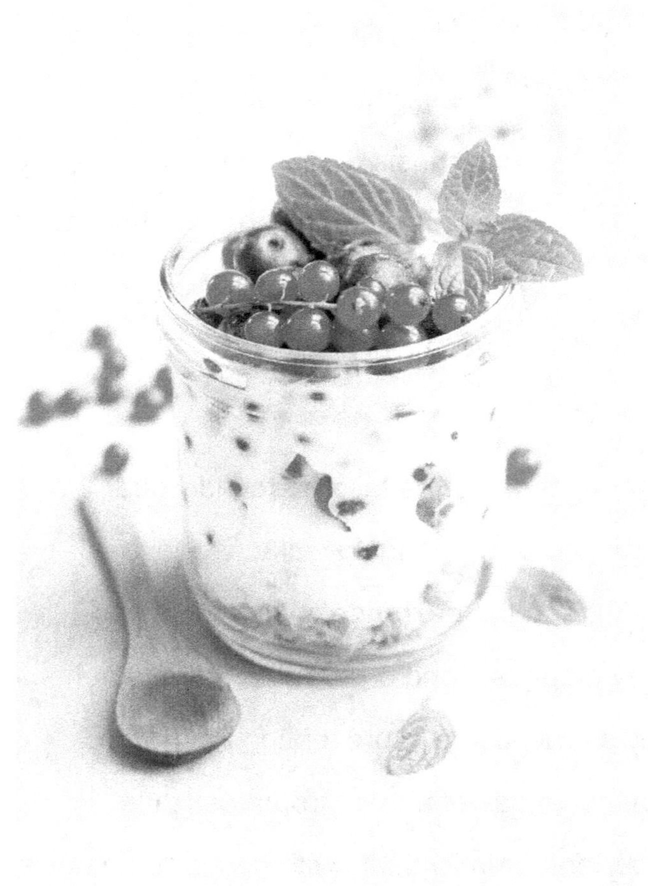

Chapter eight

The hemochromatosis diets

Dietary management is an essential component of hemochromatosis care, aiming to reduce iron absorption and maintain iron balance in individuals with this condition. Here are dietary considerations for those with hemochromatosis:

1. Limit Iron-Rich Foods:
    - Red Meat: While red meat is a good source of heme iron, individuals with hemochromatosis should moderate their intake. Choose lesser amounts and lean meats.
    - Organ Meats: Liver and other organ meats are particularly high

in iron and should be limited or
avoided.

- Shellfish: Certain shellfish, such as clams and mussels, are rich in iron and should be consumed in moderation.

2. Be Mindful of Non-Heme Iron Sources:

- Plant-Based Iron: While non-heme iron from plant sources is generally less readily absorbed than heme iron, individuals with hemochromatosis should still be mindful of their intake. Include a variety of plant-based foods but consider moderating consumption of high-iron items like fortified cereals, legumes, and spinach.

3. Limit Vitamin C Intake During Meals:

- Enhanced Absorption: Vitamin C enhances non-heme iron absorption. While vitamin C is essential for health, individuals with hemochromatosis should consider separating high-vitamin C foods or supplements from iron-rich meals to reduce iron absorption.

4. Avoid Iron Supplements Unless Prescribed:

- Caution with Supplements: Iron supplements should generally be avoided unless specifically prescribed by a healthcare professional. Excessive iron intake can exacerbate iron overload in individuals with hemochromatosis.

5. Limit Alcohol Consumption:

   - Liver Health: Alcohol can contribute to liver damage, and individuals with hemochromatosis are advised to limit or avoid alcohol consumption to protect against complications.

6. Stay Hydrated:

   - Fluids During Phlebotomy: For those undergoing phlebotomy, staying well-hydrated can make blood removal easier. Adequate hydration is generally beneficial for overall health.

7. Regular Monitoring and Individualized Plans:

   - Consult a Dietitian: Individual dietary needs can vary, and consulting a registered dietitian experienced in hemochromatosis can be beneficial. They can help create a personalized diet plan considering specific iron levels, lifestyle, and nutritional requirements.

8. Whole Grains and Calcium-Rich Foods:

    o Phytic Acid and Calcium: Foods containing phytic acid (found in whole grains and legumes) and calcium can inhibit iron absorption. Including these in the diet may help regulate iron absorption.

It's crucial for individuals with hemochromatosis to work closely with healthcare professionals and dietitians to create a balanced and sustainable dietary plan.

Regular monitoring of iron levels, along with
dietary adjustments, can help manage iron
overload effectively and improve overall
well-bein

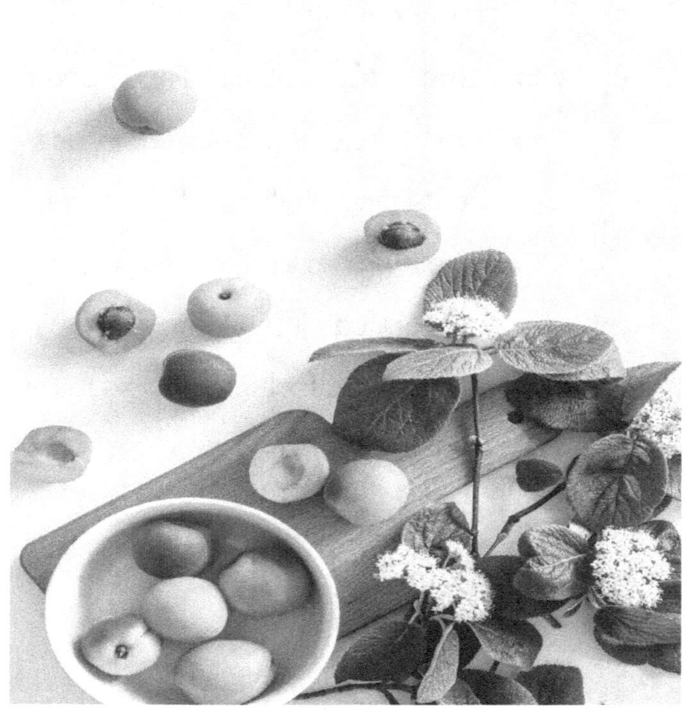

Chapter nine

Beneficial foods

In managing hemochromatosis, incorporating a balanced and nutrient-rich diet can be beneficial. While it's crucial to be mindful of iron-rich foods, there are also certain elements in a diet that can be advantageous for individuals with hemochromatosis. Here are some beneficial foods and dietary considerations:

1. Calcium-Rich Foods:
   - Dairy Products: Calcium competes with iron for absorption. Including dairy products like milk, yogurt, and cheese in your diet may help regulate iron absorption.

2. Whole Grains and Legumes:

    ○ Phytic Acid Content: Whole grains and legumes contain phytic acid, which can inhibit iron absorption. Including these foods in your diet may contribute to managing iron levels.

3. Fruits and Vegetables:

    ○ Antioxidants: Fruits and vegetables, rich in antioxidants, can support overall health. They are also low in iron, making them suitable choices for individuals with hemochromatosis.

    ○ Vitamin C: While vitamin C enhances non-heme iron absorption, its inclusion in the diet can still be beneficial. Consider consuming vitamin

C-rich fruits and vegetables

separately from iron-rich meals.

4. Lean Proteins:

   o Poultry and Fish: Lean protein

   sources like chicken and fish are

   lower in iron compared to red

   meat. Including these options can

   provide essential nutrients

   without significantly increasing

   iron intake.

5. Hydration:

   o Water and Fluids: Staying

   hydrated is important, especially

   for individuals undergoing

   phlebotomy. Well-hydrated blood

   can make the process of blood

   removal more efficient.

6. Moderation of Iron-Fortified Foods:

- Fortified Cereals and Foods: While fortified foods can contribute essential nutrients, including iron, moderation is key. Be mindful of the iron content in these products.

7. Consultation with a Dietitian:
   - Individualized Guidance: Working with a registered dietitian can provide personalized dietary guidance. They can help create a plan that considers specific iron levels, lifestyle, and nutritional needs.

8. Herbal Teas:
   - Tannins in Tea: Tannins in tea can inhibit non-heme iron absorption. Consuming herbal teas, which are typically low in

tannins, may be a suitable alternative to regular tea.

It's important to emphasize that individual responses to dietary adjustments can vary, and consulting with healthcare professionals, including dietitians, is crucial. Regular monitoring of iron levels allows for adjustments to the dietary plan as needed. A well-rounded and varied diet can contribute to overall health and help manage iron levels effectively in individuals with hemochromatosis.

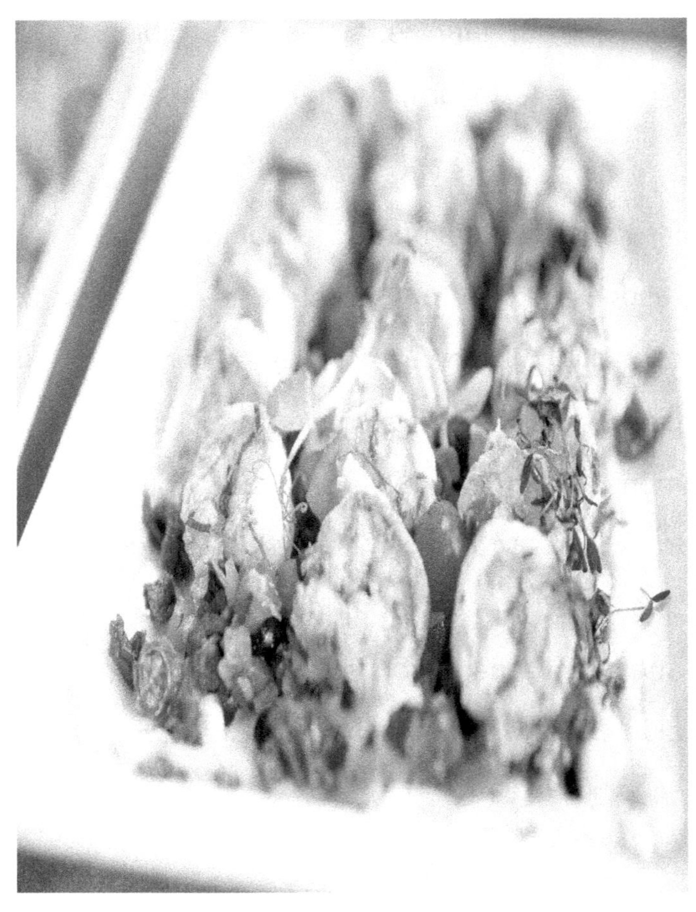

Chapter ten

Foods to avoid and a shopping list for hemochromatosis

Foods to Avoid in Hemochromatosis:

1. Red and Organ Meats:

    - Beef, lamb, pork, and organ meats are high in heme iron and should be consumed in moderation.

2. Shellfish:

    - Certain shellfish, such as clams and mussels, are rich in iron and should be limited.

3. Iron-Fortified Foods:

    - Some cereals, bread, and processed foods are fortified with iron. Check labels and choose lower-iron alternatives.

4. Vitamin C Supplements with Meals:

   o High-dose vitamin C supplements taken with iron-rich meals can enhance iron absorption. Separate vitamin C supplements from meals.

5. Alcohol:

   o Limit or avoid alcohol consumption, as it can contribute to liver damage in individuals with hemochromatosis.

6. Excessive Iron Supplements:

   o Avoid iron supplements unless prescribed by a healthcare professional to prevent iron overload.

7. High Iron Vegetables:

   o While vegetables are generally healthy, some like spinach and

other dark leafy greens have
higher iron content. Moderation is
advised.

8. Uncooked Seafood:

    o Raw or undercooked seafood can
      pose risks and should be
      avoided.

Hemochromatosis-Friendly Shopping List:

1. Lean Proteins:

    o Skinless poultry (chicken, turkey).

    o Fish (especially varieties lower in
      iron like salmon and trout).

2. Dairy Products:

    o Low-fat or fat-free milk.

    o Yogurt.

    o Cheese (in moderation).

3. Fruits:

- Apples.

- Berries (blueberries, strawberries).

- Citrus fruits (oranges, grapefruits).

4. Vegetables:

   - Broccoli.

   - Cauliflower.

   - Bell peppers.

5. Whole Grains:

   - Brown rice.

   - Quinoa.

   - Oats.

6. Legumes:

   - Lentils.

   - Chickpeas.

   - Black beans.

7. Nuts and Seeds:

   - Almonds.

- o Sunflower seeds.

  - o Pumpkin seeds.

8. Herbal Teas:

  - o Chamomile tea.

  - o Peppermint tea.

9. Hydration:

  - o Water.

10. Calcium-Rich Foods:

  - o Low-fat or fat-free dairy products.

  - o Tofu (calcium-set).

Remember, individual dietary needs vary, and it's essential to tailor the diet to personal health conditions and preferences. Consultation with a healthcare professional or a registered dietitian can provide personalized guidance and ensure that nutritional needs are met while managing iron levels effectively.

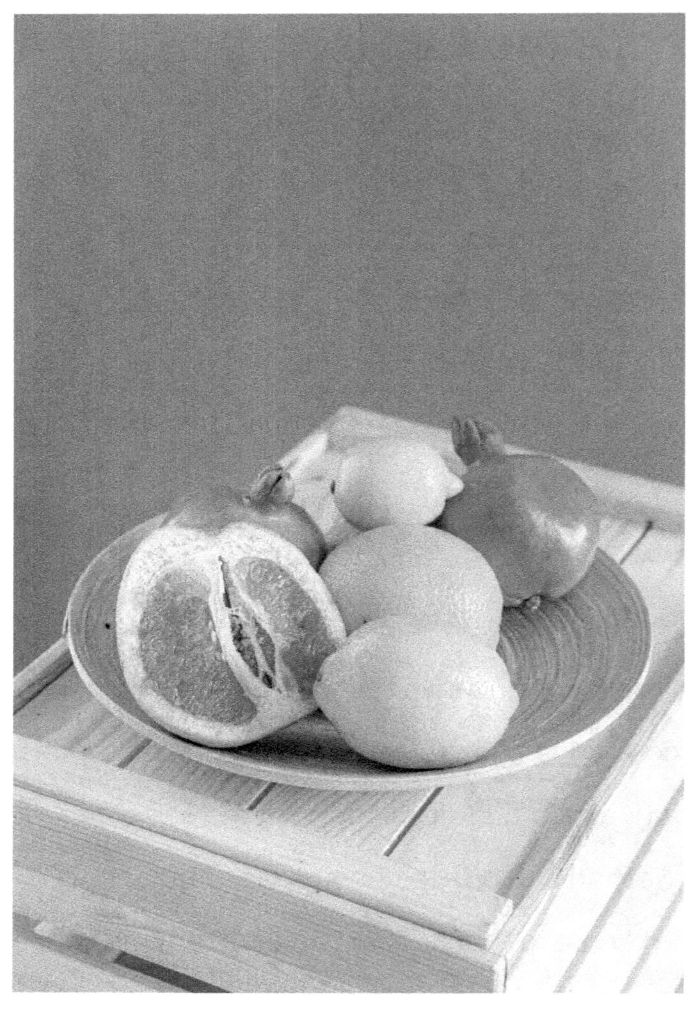

Chapter eleven

Meal plan and time table for hemochromatosis

Creating a meal plan for hemochromatosis involves balancing nutrient intake while managing iron levels. It's important to emphasize moderation in consuming iron-rich foods and consider the timing of meals. Below is a sample meal plan along with a suggested timetable for individuals with hemochromatosis:

Sample Meal Plan:

Breakfast (8:00 AM):

- Oatmeal made with water or low-fat milk.
- Fresh berries (blueberries, strawberries).
- Toast with almond butter.

Mid-Morning Snack (10:30 AM):

- Greek yogurt with sliced almonds.
- Apple slices.

Lunch (12:30 PM):

- salad of grilled chicken or tofu topped with cherry tomatoes, mixed greens, and vinaigrette dressing.
- Quinoa or brown rice on the side.
- Steamed broccoli.

Afternoon Snack (3:00 PM):

- Hummus with carrot and cucumber sticks.
- Handful of grapes.

Dinner (6:30 PM):

- Baked salmon or trout.

- Sweet potato or roasted cauliflower.

- Mixed green salad with olive oil dressing.

Evening Snack (8:30 PM):

- A small handful of nuts (almonds or walnuts).

- Herbal tea (chamomile or peppermint).

Tips for Hemochromatosis Meal Planning:

1. Hydration:

   - Drink plenty of water throughout the day. Staying hydrated can support overall health and facilitate blood removal during phlebotomy.

2. Calcium-Rich Foods:
   - Include low-fat or fat-free dairy products, tofu, and leafy greens to help regulate iron absorption.

3. Limit Vitamin C with Iron-Rich Meals:
   - Consume vitamin C-rich foods separately from iron-rich meals to moderate iron absorption.

4. Lean Proteins:
   - Choose lean protein sources like poultry, fish, and plant-based proteins.

5. Whole Grains:
   - Opt for whole grains like quinoa, brown rice, and oats to provide essential nutrients without excessive iron.

6. Vegetables and Fruits:

    o   Include a variety of colorful

        vegetables and fruits for

        antioxidants and other essential

        nutrients.

7. Monitor Portion Sizes:

    o   Be mindful of portion sizes,

        especially with iron-rich foods.

8. Avoid Alcohol:

    o   Limit or avoid alcohol to protect

        against liver damage.

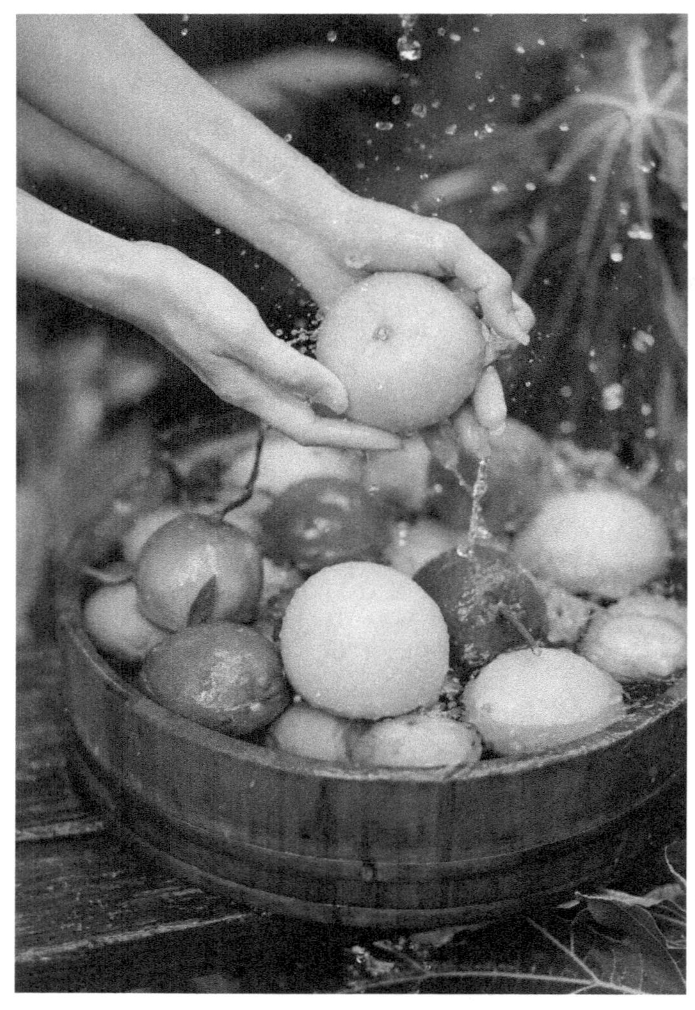

Chapter twelve

Soups and Salads

Creating soups and salads for individuals with hemochromatosis involves incorporating ingredients that are nutrient-dense and balanced while being mindful of iron content. Here are some ideas for soups and salads suitable for those with hemochromatosis:

Soups:

1. Vegetable Broth Soup:

    o   Ingredients: Low-iron vegetables (carrots, celery, zucchini), low-sodium vegetable broth, herbs (parsley, thyme), quinoa or barley.

2. Chicken and Vegetable Soup:

    o   Ingredients: Lean chicken, low-iron vegetables (green

beans, carrots, spinach),
low-sodium chicken broth, herbs
(rosemary, dill), and whole-grain
noodles.

3. Lentil Soup:

   o Ingredients: Lentils, low-iron
   vegetables (tomatoes, onions,
   carrots), low-sodium vegetable
   broth, cumin, coriander, and a
   squeeze of lemon.

4. Mushroom and Barley Soup:

   o Ingredients: Mushrooms, barley,
   low-sodium vegetable broth,
   onions, garlic, and thyme.

Salads:

1. Spinach and Strawberry Salad:

- Ingredients: Fresh spinach, strawberries, walnuts, feta cheese (in moderation), and a balsamic vinaigrette dressing.

2. Chickpea Salad:

   - Ingredients: Chickpeas, cherry tomatoes, cucumber, red onion, parsley, olive oil, and lemon juice.

3. Quinoa and Vegetable Salad:

   - Ingredients: Quinoa, bell peppers, cherry tomatoes, cucumber, feta cheese (in moderation), and a lemon-tahini dressing.

4. Grilled Chicken Caesar Salad (moderation):

   - Ingredients: Grilled chicken breast, romaine lettuce, cherry

tomatoes, croutons (limited), and
a low-iron Caesar dressing.

Tips for Hemochromatosis-Friendly Soups and Salads:

1. Iron-Aware Ingredients:

    - Choose low-iron vegetables like leafy greens, carrots, and bell peppers.
    - Be mindful of ingredient portions, especially those high in iron, such as meats and certain cheeses.

2. Limit Iron-Rich Proteins:

    - Opt for lean proteins like grilled chicken, tofu, or legumes in moderation.

3. Herbs and Spices:

    - Use herbs and spices for flavor instead of iron-rich seasonings.

Examples include garlic, thyme, rosemary, and lemon.

4. Homemade Dressings:
   - Make your own dressings using olive oil, vinegar, and herbs to control ingredients and iron content.

5. Hydration:
   - Soups can contribute to hydration. Choose broths and clear soups to stay hydrated.

6. Variety and Color:
   - Include a variety of colorful vegetables to ensure a diverse nutrient intake.

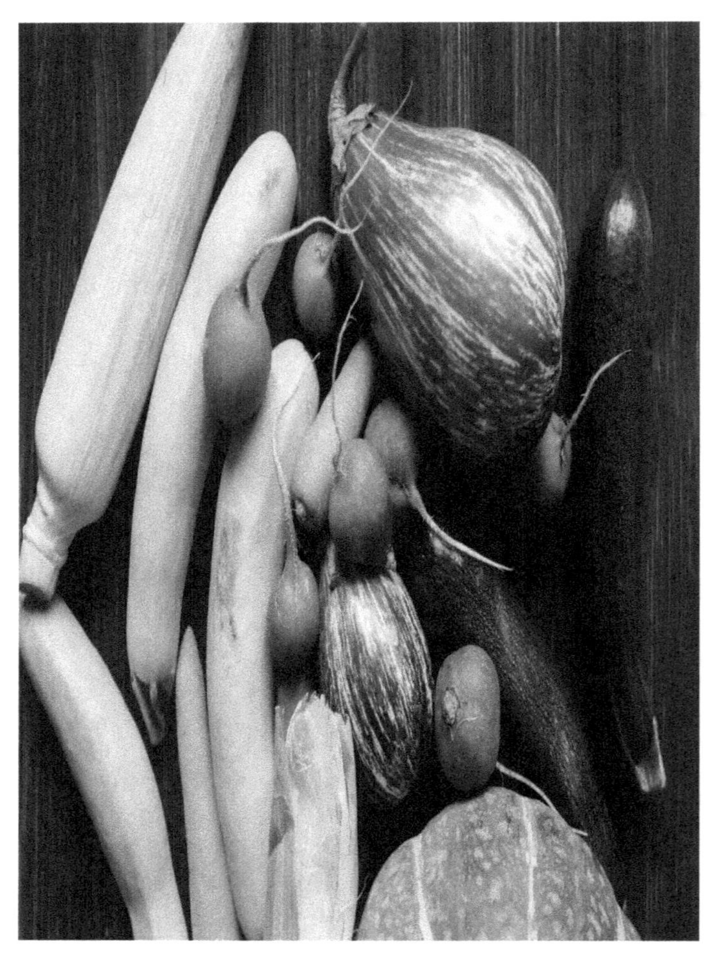

Chapter thirteen

Desserts

Creating desserts for individuals with hemochromatosis involves focusing on options that are lower in iron and mindful of other dietary considerations. Here are some dessert ideas suitable for those with hemochromatosis:

1. Fruit Salad with Mint:

- Ingredients:
    - Assorted fresh fruits (e.g., berries, melons, kiwi)
    - Fresh mint leaves
    - Optional: A drizzle of balsamic glaze or honey
- Instructions:
    - Combine fresh fruits in a bowl.
    - Garnish with mint leaves.

- Optionally, drizzle with a small amount of balsamic glaze or honey for added sweetness.

2. Yogurt Parfait:

- Ingredients:
    - Greek yogurt (low-fat or non-fat)
    - Mixed berries
    - Granola (low-iron variety)
    - Optional: Nuts (in moderation)
- Instructions:
    - In a glass or dish, arrange mixed berries and Greek yogurt.
    - Sprinkle with granola and, if desired, add a small amount of nuts.

3. Chia Seed Pudding:

- Ingredients:

- - Chia seeds
  - Almond milk (or any non-dairy milk)
  - Vanilla extract
  - Fresh fruit for topping
- Instructions:
  - Mix chia seeds with almond milk and vanilla extract.
  - Refrigerate until the mixture thickens (usually a few hours or overnight).
  - Top with fresh fruit before serving.

4. Sorbet:

- Ingredients:
  - Mixed fruit sorbet (store-bought or homemade)
  - Fresh mint leaves for garnish

- Instructions:
    - Scoop sorbet into individual servings.
    - Garnish with fresh mint leaves.

5. Baked Apples:

- Ingredients:
    - Apples (choose low-iron varieties)
    - Cinnamon
    - Chopped nuts (in moderation)
- Instructions:
    - Core apples and sprinkle with cinnamon.
    - Optionally, fill the center with chopped nuts.
    - Bake until tender.

6. Banana Nice Cream:

- Ingredients:
    - Ripe bananas
    - Vanilla extract
    - Optional: Nut butter (in moderation)
- Instructions:
    - Freeze ripe bananas.
    - Blend frozen bananas with a splash of vanilla extract until smooth.
    - Optionally, swirl in a small amount of nut butter.

Tips for Hemochromatosis-Friendly Desserts:

1. Portion Control:

- o   Pay attention to portion sizes to prevent consuming too many calories.

2. Moderation with Nuts and Seeds:

   - o   If including nuts or seeds, do so in moderation due to their iron content.

3. Natural Sweeteners:

   - o   Use natural sweeteners sparingly, such as honey or maple syrup.

4. Hydration:

   - o   Incorporate desserts with high water content, like fruit salads and sorbets, to support hydration.

Conclusion

In conclusion, crafting a cookbook tailored to individuals with hemochromatosis involves a thoughtful blend of nutrient-rich recipes that focus on managing iron levels while maintaining a satisfying and diverse culinary experience. From hearty soups and salads to refreshing desserts, the emphasis is on incorporating low-iron alternatives and balancing key ingredients to meet nutritional needs without exacerbating iron overload.

The suggested meal plans and recipes provide a foundation for individuals with hemochromatosis to navigate their dietary choices, promoting wellness and preventing complications associated with excess iron. By prioritizing lean proteins, whole grains, and a colorful array of fruits and vegetables, these recipes cater to a balanced and enjoyable approach to nutrition.

Furthermore, the cookbook encourages mindfulness in food selection, portion control, and strategic pairing of ingredients to optimize nutrient absorption. The inclusion of hydration-focused desserts and the incorporation of natural sweeteners contribute to a well-rounded and health-conscious culinary experience.

It's essential for individuals with hemochromatosis to consult with healthcare professionals and dietitians for personalized guidance. Regular monitoring of iron levels and adherence to dietary recommendations outlined in this cookbook can empower individuals to manage their condition effectively, promoting a healthy and fulfilling lifestyle. This cookbook stands as a practical resource, combining culinary delight with nutritional wisdom to enhance the well-being of those navigating the challenges of hemochromatosis.